MEAL PLANNING ON A BUDGET

Save Money on Groceries, Master Meal Prep, & Reduce Food Waste to Reach Financial Freedom

JEN SMITH

Copyright © 2018 Jen Smith, Modern Frugality & Saving With Spunk

All rights reserved.

ISBN-13: 978-1977046574

YOUR FREE GIFT

As a thank you for purchasing this book I wanted to give you some extra resources to help you along your food journey.

The Meal Planning on a Budget Bundle is a free workbook that includes:

- Printable weekly menu
- Printable monthly menu
- Categorized list of 75 of my favorite food blogs for recipes
- 20 Items to always keep in your pantry and what emergency meals you can make with them

It's all free for you and available at: modernfrugality.com/mealplanbundle

And for a complete list of all my recommendations in this book be sure to visit: modernfrugality.com/recommendations-from-meal-planning-on-a-budget

To Travis, thank you for your support, encouragement, and eating whatever I put in front of you.

CONTENTS

	Introduction: You Need a Meal Plan	1
1	Meal Planning for Fun and Profit	5
2	How to Save Money on Groceries Without Losing Your Soul	18
3	Meal Preppers	36
4	Reduce, Reuse, Eat	46
5	Sample Meal Plan with Prep Guide	59
6	Keeping it Real Sustainable	67

INTRODUCTION: YOU NEED A MEAL PLAN

For most of my life I've had a sordid relationship with food. I grew up with a working mom and saw the drive-thru at McDonalds a lot. I learned how to cook by grabbing a bag from the freezer, cutting it open, and pouring it into a skillet.

I don't remember any shopping lists or meals made from scratch and I was always a little chubbier than friends my age. So when I went to college and discovered that I actually had to buy food for myself, I went to the grocery store and realized I had no clue what I was doing.

Now, if grocery shopping had been a class in high school, I would've rocked it like a pro. But it wasn't, and if you don't learn this stuff at home, you don't learn it. And what 17-year-old wants to sit down with their parent and learn to plan meals?

When I got married I found myself in bed with another

person who wandered around lost in the grocery store. We were two typical millennials who loved to eat out and had never taken a home economics course. And, to top it off, had completely opposite food preferences.

But we had made it our mission to pay off the almost $78,000 of debt we had as quickly as possible. I knew that in order to do that, we'd have to stop eating out and find common ground in the kitchen.

More than that, we needed to be strategic about grocery shopping. If left to our own devices and hanger (hunger + anger), we'd spend as much on groceries as we did going to restaurants.

Since I enjoy planning, I took up the challenge of getting our grocery budget as low as possible. And I got pretty good at it.

So good, in fact, that one week I only spent $14 on groceries. No lie!

In my first book, The No-Spend Challenge Guide, I sang the praises of meal planning and prepping as a way to eliminate extra trips to the grocery store, thus eliminating more impulse buys. I wanted to write another practical guide to not only help you save money on groceries but to transform your relationship with food spending.

It's easy to find apps and products that will plan your meals one week at a time or focus on meal planning for fitness, but coupled with the cost of purchasing pricey ingredients, they end up costing you around the same amount they save you.

I searched Amazon high and low for a book like this and I couldn't find it!

There are full books on the topics of meal planning and prepping for weight loss or shopping at Aldi. There is no all-inclusive guide to saving money on groceries by shopping smart, meal planning, prepping, and reducing food waste.

This book is designed to:

- Teach you to meal plan efficiently.
- Help you save money at the grocery store.
- Teach you to meal prep like a pro, making cooking throughout the week faster.
- Teach you how to make foods last longer so you can stop throwing money in the garbage.

This is not some basic "talk at you" guide that you could get if you searched Google. This is carefully crafted information that I hope will be your launching pad to master meal planning, grocery shopping, meal prepping, and cooking through your busy week.

How Much Money Will This Book Save Me?

I can't tell you that. I don't know how much money you spend on groceries. But I can tell you I wrote this book for beginners. I wrote it for people who are working on getting out of debt and realize they need to cut their food budget in order to succeed.

For some people this information will seem like "common sense drivel," but after talking to a lot of millennials about this subject, I've found that "common sense" isn't common anymore.

I didn't know most of this stuff three years ago. Heck, some of it I learned while researching for this book. Don't assume everyone starts from the same point and don't feel guilty if this is all new to you.

You'll get more out of this book if you're beginning your journey to financial independence, but I think even seasoned frugal shoppers can learn something new. However, if you've been shopping at Aldi for years or couponing so hard they put you on TV, save your money for another book.

So if you're ready to take a new approach to spending on food then keep reading. It won't be easy at first, but it's simple. I've filled this book with as many high-impact tips as I could find and I know you'll find new information and helpful reminders in every chapter.

[1]
MEAL PLANNING FOR FUN AND PROFIT

American households throw away $640 worth of food every year. That's a new smartphone every year, or dinner at a nice restaurant once a month. And in the last four decades, food waste has increased over 50%. Oh, and we also consume more calories than the average person did 40 years ago.

I know ya gotta eat, but the amount Americans (especially millennials) spend on eating out and wasting food is embarrassing.

There are so many methods to start meal planning, from complete DIY to having every meal completely done for you. Paying for this service is absolutely worth it for some people (and we'll talk about it later) but everyone should know how to execute the basic task of meal planning.

But meal planning isn't just picking recipes and compiling a grocery list. To really overhaul your food budget, you have to look at every aspect of your food, from how much you buy and where it's stored to where its final destination is.

We make a big fuss about meal planning and saving on groceries in the personal finance world, but we don't talk as much about strategies to make sure the food gets used, stays fresh and edible, or works for you.

If you want a life and finances that are holistically healthy, then food needs to be your top priority in discretionary spending.

Meal Planning Vs. Meal Kits

Sometimes when I talk about meal planning, people think I'm referring to meal kits mailed to your home from companies like Blue Apron, Hello Fresh, and Marley Spoon. These companies may claim to be cheaper than grocery shopping but I think we can all agree that it depends on what you're buying.

Meal kits have unique recipes with exotic ingredients that, if you're buying full sizes, do add up. Even with discount coupons and free shipping, you're still paying about $10 per meal. And then you still have to do dishes. Meal planning allows you to overlap ingredients, sub out for less expensive ones, and alter quantities to allow for leftovers.

If your creativity is in a slump or you're just starting out in the kitchen and really want to try one, my friend came up with a technique to stretch meal kits: You can see the recipes being delivered to you online before you get the ingredients. Buy extra of the cheapest/most filling ingredients in the recipes and add them in to assure leftovers the next day.

Ultimately, meal kits are not going to help you cut your food budget because it limits your flexibility in the grocery store. But they're not inherently evil and I've liked them when I've tried them.

Why Meal Plan?

You probably already have an answer to this question or you wouldn't be reading this book right now. You want to eat out less, eat healthier, save money, and use more of those pantry items you've been hoarding. And there are probably 100 more reasons (rough guess) that you haven't even considered.

I'd guess that most people hate meal planning, but I love it. I love it way more than cooking, albeit I'm also way better at it than cooking.

Having a meal plan means you can make an accurate grocery list that ensures you have what you need and accounts for substitutions ahead of time. It means fewer trips to the grocery store, less chance to be tempted by "off-list" items, and less time waiting in checkout lines.

For those of us who don't consider ourselves home chefs, meal planning helps you practice the art of cooking (a skill Americans are quickly losing) and eat a variety of meals from different cuisines. You can tailor healthy meals no matter how busy your day is because you're prepared.

And my favorite, avoiding the dreaded "What's for dinner?" question.

I used to rely on premade meals, ending up with random impulse buys in my pantry or junk food my hips didn't need. The simple act of consistent meal planning took me from Trader Joe's wanderer to grocery store crusader and I hope it'll help you do the same.

Getting Started

For people who don't have the "planning gene," I'm sure all of this sounds horrible. You're a "fly by the seat of your pants" type of person, I get it, but hear me out. Meal planning doesn't have to be a rigid set of limitations you adhere to week-in and week-out. You can make a plan as flexible as you are.

After years of doing this I've found that planning four to five dinners a week is my sweet spot. Yep, you read right, no more than five. We don't eat out the other days of the week, but things do come up, we'll go to a friend's house or eat cereal for dinner. And some recipes make lots of leftovers.

Even if you only have 30 minutes, you can pick five recipes with similar ingredients and call it a plan. If that's what you need to get started, then awesome! I'm proud of you for starting.

The tips in this book help you build on that to maximize time and money-saving efforts. But it's important to realize you can't implement everything all at once, you should start small and work up from there.

In order to make meal planning a sustainable practice and, eventually, an automatic habit, here are the steps to take to build your weekly meal plan.

How to Meal Plan in Five Easy Steps

1. Take Inventory

Restaurants use the acronym FIFO: First In, First Out. They use the produce they have before they use the new stuff, which is how they save money and stay profitable. In order for your kitchen to stay profitable, it makes sense to adopt the same rule.

Take a look at your fridge and pantry and **write down five things you want to use this week based on what's going bad and/or the FIFO rule.** You can pick more or fewer items but you don't need to take a full inventory of your kitchen every week, five will do.

Most grocery store vegetables will last a few weeks but some have a shorter shelf life. If you have a long list, order it in priority based on what's going bad first. You may not be able to get to everything and you might have to throw something out. Mourn the loss and do better next time. (RIP celery, literally every time I buy it.)

2. Look at Sales

When you get that weekly ad in the mail or newspaper, you should look at it instead of tossing it directly into the recycling. But you should know a few things about these flyers before you make your list.

Not everything advertised in your grocery ad is actually on sale. Yep, it's unfortunate but true. A large portion of the flyer is advertising space the store has sold to product manufacturers, leaving the "featured" price the same as any other day.

Stores will also run BOGO deals or two for $5 deals, and many times these aren't true BOGO deals. They make you think you need to buy two items when really you can buy one and get the sale. For some reason I see this all the time with avocados. The signs say "10 avocados for $10" when you can actually get one avocado for a dollar. So check the fine print to make sure.

Rules of thumb when finding sales: Ignore brand name products in ads and read the fine print on "quantity" sales. Advertisements for fresh and store brand products are usually legit sales. They're usually seasonal produce and products so it's not hard to identify them. The ad might also state "new low price" or "originally $X.99" when the item is truly on sale.

Once you've scanned the flyer, add three to five sales you want to take advantage of to the bottom of your inventory list. If it's longer than that, you can rate them in order of best deal or what you're craving most.

3. Evaluate Your Calendar

Which nights do you have knitting club? Which nights are you working late or side hustling? Is the boss buying lunch on Friday? Do you have a wedding this weekend? Everything on your schedule affects your meal plan.

Know how many dinners and lunches you need for the week and the amount of time you have to make them. I like to average five dinners in my plan but if we go to my in-laws on Sunday I know I'll take leftovers home, so it could be a three dinner week. (#LearnToLoveLeftovers)

And as your schedule changes, this might be the week you have time to make that intricate recipe you've been eyeing and next week might be a five freezer meals kinda week. Too many recipes, not enough for leftovers, and recipes you don't have time to make are the downfall of a meal plan.

You may also want to add breakfast and lunch to your meal plan based on your schedule, family size, and dietary needs. We keep breakfast real simple, usually opting for cereal, a protein shake, or overnight oats if I'm feeling fancy. Lunch is always leftovers and I have backup food if there aren't enough leftovers for a full meal.

And it may seem like common sense but you should plan when you're next going to the grocery store so you have enough meals to last you until then. Hopefully you'll have a set day of the week that you shop, but if your schedule doesn't permit going on that day you'll need to adjust your meal plan accordingly.

4. Select Recipes

All right, here's the big one. With your inventory priorities, sale items, and schedule assembled, you can take to the internet and cookbooks to find recipes that meet your time and ingredient requirements.

When selecting a week's worth of recipes we're not trying to be Julia Child over here. Pick simple recipes and get creative when you know you have time. It's unlikely you'll be able to include all of your desired inventory or sale items, so prioritize by using what you have first and incorporating sales where you can.

If you haven't already, visit the resource page mentioned in the front of the book to download the free meal planning bundle. I've listed and categorized my 75 favorite websites for easy, budget-friendly recipes and you'll get free printable menus.

Selecting recipes doesn't have to just happen when you're planning, it can happen any time. Whenever I have a few minutes to kill or I get an idea for a recipe, I'll browse food blogs or search ingredients for the best take on what I'm craving. Pinterest is great but good ol' Google is fantastic too. I also get cookbooks from the library and look for those short cooking videos that are all over Facebook.

Facebook pages to follow for awesome cooking videos:

- Tasty
- Spoon University
- 12 Tomatoes
- Struggle Meals

I compile all of these ideas on Pinterest. Not only is Pinterest a recipe searcher's paradise, it's a great way to organize your recipes. The simplest method (and the way I still do it) is to have two boards: "New Recipes" and "Tried & Loved."

Whether it's a random dinner picture on Instagram or I'm looking for new recipes with potatoes because they're celebrating their third consecutive week on sale, I save a bunch of interesting recipes to limit my active meal planning time. All these new recipes go on the "New Recipes" board. Once I make them, if I don't like it I delete it, and if I do like it I transfer it to "Tried & Loved."

It's nice to have all my go-to recipes on a separate board for easy reference. When I see butternut squash on sale, I know the first thing I'm going to make is Gimme Some Oven's yummy squash soup that I've loved for years. I'm not going to waste time searching for new squash recipes until it's the end of winter and my husband is begging me to stop making him that soup. When you build up an arsenal of loved recipes, it makes meal planning much faster.

If Pinterest isn't your thing, there are other free apps that can store recipes from the internet. Paprika is a free recipe-storing app with an intuitive user interface, easy navigation, and smart grocery lists. Pepperplate is a similar free app that's not as intuitive but is great for the iPad, if that's your preferred device.

Another way to make recipe selection faster and easier is assigning each night of the week a theme. Typical themes are Meatless Monday, Taco Tuesday, Water Chestnut Wednesday, whatever works for you. We used to do a frozen pizza every Wednesday (one of the reasons we got away with a five-recipe meal plan), but we're trying to minimize our carbs now so we're trying new things.

You can always change it up if you hate it. Be flexible and you'll be successful.

Once you've chosen your recipes and assigned them a day, put your menu on the fridge so you can easily reference it. I started out with a scrap paper menu but found a magnetic dry erase menu for $5 — an investment

I highly recommend. You can see my recommendation in the resource guide for this book.

5. Make Your Grocery List

Now you have everything you need to make your grocery list. This is another process I start during the week because toilet paper and deodorant never show up in recipes. I prefer scrap paper, usually the back of envelopes from credit card solicitations, but there are apps if you prefer.

*Pro Tip: Shout out to my editor for this tip, if you use a scrap envelope for your list you can put your coupons and cash in it!

The advantage of using an app is you can have an updated list of what's in your pantry without having to write it down every week. Finished off that bottle of dried dill? Erase it from the pantry list and move it to this week's shopping list, or don't, because how often do you use dill? List Ease is a good free app for that.

Regardless of where you keep your list, make your list while in the kitchen so you can easily check how much you have to determine how much you need. Only put things on your list that you're out or nearly out of. When reducing your grocery spending and food waste there's no room for "wishful thinking" on the grocery list.

Don't be afraid to substitute ingredients. Something that will save you a ton of money and save your cabinets from clutter is substituting ingredients in recipes. Cooking is science, sometimes substituting is as easy as subtracting a few tablespoons or adding some vinegar.

Allrecipes has this nifty substitutions guide for many ingredients. My rule is I won't buy a random ingredient like cake flour, chervil, or arrowroot starch just for it to sit in my cabinet unused if I can substitute it with a commonly used item I already have. It saves me money and maintains my minimalist kitchen.

Last but not least, account for any meals you want to double to make an extra freezer meal. I don't make one every week but I always have one or two waiting in my freezer for busy weeks or when something unplanned comes up.

And there you go, that's the gist of meal planning for budget purposes. You could stop here but you'd be missing out on so many more opportunities to save money on food. That's the 101, now let me take you on an advanced journey into meal planning.

Meal Planning 201 - Batch Planning

Once you've been doing this for a while, you'll have a good idea of the recipes you like, a stockpile of freezer meals, and be pretty tired of giving up hours every Sunday to prep stuff. When you have reached this stage, you're ready to graduate to batch planning.

Batch meal planning is making a schedule for weeks at a time. I suggest starting with two weeks, then stepping up to four weeks. I wouldn't plan for more than four weeks at a time because life can change so rapidly.

I'll confess to you that I can't get to meal planning every Sunday. Sometimes we're busy and I can't make time for it. Sometimes I'll get through planning and shopping and take a nap instead of prepping. Batch planning means you don't have to carve out time every week to plan.

It also helps you get ahead on prepping ingredients for the following weeks, cutting down on prep time later on, and reducing food waste. If there's a recipe you want to make this week that includes two carrots, you can schedule a recipe for next week that uses four more and reduce the number you'll have to freeze.

Another option in batch planning is picking a certain cuisine to focus on for a few weeks so you can master those flavors and cooking techniques. I prefer variety but for you budding chefs, this would be a great way to master a cuisine quickly.

If you're human, you're going to want to graduate to batch planning at some point. It's easier to maintain but it's daunting to start out with. Get familiar with weekly and biweekly meal planning before you jump into four-week plans.

In Chapter 5, I've included a sample four-week meal plan with meal prep guide. You'll see suggestions for breakfasts, lunches, and five dinners each week. It isn't a completely cohesive meal plan (in order to show menus from sales in different seasons) but it has the same variety I would use in a batch meal plan.

The one downside to batch planning is that you can't see the ads in the future. Some stores put out their ads two weeks early but you won't find them three or four weeks in advance. You can search for archives of your store's ads to see what was on sale this time last year and get an idea of what will be on sale in the future. And when in doubt, you're always safe with in-season produce and special buys.

Action Steps:

- Take an inventory of what you already have in the fridge.
- Look up recipes using those ingredients.
- Start storing recipes on your Pinterest boards or app.

[2]

HOW TO SAVE MONEY ON GROCERIES WITHOUT LOSING YOUR SOUL

Now that you have your menu and grocery list ready, it's time to get the deals. You'll probably be familiar with some of these methods and others not so much. I've only included the strategies I think are the most effective in saving money.

You may think you have to learn some extreme couponing techniques to make efforts worth your while but it's not the most efficient (or healthiest) way to save money. Following a few practical rules will help you save money wherever and whenever you're at the grocery store.

At the end of this chapter I've included a guide to shopping at Aldi, which I've found has saved me more money than any method I've tried. Not everyone has an Aldi or comparable store near them so I've laid out all the good tips to make this chapter helpful for the majority of people. But if you do have an Aldi near you and you're hesitant to make the switch, I've got you covered.

Change is Good

We have a variety of grocery stores in my city, from artisanal markets with $20 jars of local pickles to stereotypically healthy stores. We have bulk stores, membership stores, stores where people bring your groceries to your car for you and stores more sketchy on the inside than their dark, empty parking lot.

As someone who doesn't like change, I was hesitant to try a store that wasn't the one I was brought up with. But I knew, for the sake of my budget, I needed to see what else was out there. And I'm glad I did.

I shop primarily at Aldi now and, while its selection is limited, its prices are unbeatable. I've been shopping there for so long now I know how to change my recipes based on what they carry. If you have an Aldi nearby I highly recommend you try it out.

But I can't get everything at Aldi. For those items, I don't just go running back to my old money-sucking grocery store (that's really what it feels like when I shop there now). Instead, I buy some groceries on Amazon. I also shop at small ethnic stores. It's mostly Asian markets in my area but you can easily find Middle Eastern and Hispanic markets with a quick Google search.

If you don't have an Aldi near you, then farmer's markets, CSAs, and produce stands are cheap too. It might seem like a lot of work to go to a bunch of different places for food, so keep a small cooler in your trunk and just make a pit stop when you're nearby.

Shopping at these "off the beaten path" stores doesn't just save you money, it opens your kitchen up to a whole new world of flavor.

My final suggestion in changing how you shop is to think outside the store. U-Pick farms are cheap for picking your own produce and farmers will make trades between farms to increase the variety of produce each has available.

Oh, and you can also grow your own food if you're good at that. But don't spend a lot of money finding out if you have a green thumb or not. Pick an easy vegetable to grow (based on your climate) and if you succeed with that one, add more.

Obey the List

The list is law at the grocery store. When you get bummed out by that, remember that you make the grocery list, and the list is just keeping your inner child from making all the wrong decisions. There might be a few tantrums but you make the list because you care.

You don't take a road trip without Google Maps and you shouldn't make a grocery trip without a grocery list. So first, actually remember to bring your list!

Only put items in your cart that are on the list. If you see something new you want to try, that doesn't mean you can't try it, just put it on the list for next week and see if you still want it. You may have even planned a whole meal around it by then.

Every time you put something in your cart, keep a running calculation of your bill. No need to calculate tax—hopefully you'll fill your cart with lots of nontaxable foods. Keeping track lets you know if you have enough left in the grocery budget for that bottle of wine you deserve—as a reward for staying under budget!

Use Science!

Food is technically a means to a scientific end. You need certain nutrients to keep your body going so you don't die. Understanding this science can help you consume as little as possible and still feel great.

Foods high in fiber (such as beans, peas, and broccoli) provide volume in your stomach making you feel full for longer. Protein (like meat, eggs, oats, and Greek yogurt) influences hormones that tell your brain you're full. Healthy fats (such as nuts and avocado) decrease appetite and increase fullness.

Incorporating more of these nutrients into your meal planning and pantry will help you eat less, stretch your recipes, and spend less in the grocery store.

Stretch Your Recipe

Stretching your recipes means adding a cheap grain or produce to extend the pricier ingredients. Like adding a side of roasted sweet potatoes to chicken or mixing leftover veggies with rice (or my favorite, barley). They're also great to add on the side when you have leftovers but not enough to make a full lunch for the next day.

Some of my favorite cheap staples include:

- Rice
- Eggs
- Pasta
- Cabbage
- Dried Beans
- White Potatoes
- Sweet Potatoes

If you're looking to maximize the healthiness, shredded cabbage makes a great alternative to rice or noodles, eggs and beans are great vegetarian sources of protein, and sweet potatoes are chock-full of healthy nutrients.

Another thing to think about is government subsidies on food. Ever wonder why the unhealthy stuff is so much cheaper than healthy food? The top four foods the government subsidizes are corn, wheat, soybeans, and rice. Anything with these ingredients can be sold for way cheap because the government is paying farmers to grow them.

Views about subsidized agriculture aside, taking advantage of these subsidies in small amounts won't hurt your health and can greatly help your budget.

Only Buy Deep Discount Sale Meat

If you're going to eat meat, the easiest way to save money is to only buy it when it's on mega sale. You can look back at weekly ads for your grocery store to get an idea of the lowest sale price and how often it goes on sale for that price.

So when you see that price, you'll know it's the right time to buy and you'll also know how much to buy to last you through to the next sale. Aside from chicken, this rule will probably reduce the amount of meat you buy. When you buy in bulk you'll see how much more expensive meat is than grains, even when on sale.

I've been a vegetarian for almost a decade and it has saved me so much money. It's not for everyone but when I compare the prices of vegetarian meals and dishes to their counterparts at grocery stores and restaurants, I'm continually reminded it's a frugal win.

I was shocked the day my meat-loving husband turned down my offer to buy him ground beef burgers because he saw how much cheaper my veggie burgers were.

But you don't have to give up meat to be frugal. Chicken is a budget friendly and versatile way to keep meat on your menu, especially if you buy whole chicken and take it off the bone yourself.

You can stretch your sale meat out by using it as a mixture in dishes versus as the main event. You can still enjoy the occasional steak but it'll be much more "occasional" and special when you have it.

If you're committed to keeping red meat in your diet, stick to the cheapest cuts of pork and beef. Belly pork, pork shoulder, ham hock, brisket, and skirt steak can be reasonably affordable when on sale.

Buy In Season

It's hard to tell but not all produce is grown year-round. Summer crops like bell peppers, blueberries, cherries, and tomatoes don't grow in colder months like grapefruit, kiwi, potatoes, and winter squashes do.

But you don't have to worry about seasonality when you're shopping, the grocery store will tell you. Sales are usually on produce that's in season so all you have to do is meal plan accordingly.

Use Your Freezer

Your freezer should be stocked at all times.

Whenever produce is out of season it's sure to be cheaper in the freezer section. Frozen pizzas are great emergency meals and frozen meat is cheaper than fresh.

You can make freezer meals with on-sale produce, freeze ingredients to save for later, and, not to mention, frozen fruit is a great snack in the summer.

Another perk: store-bought frozen fruits and veggies retain all (if not more) of their nutritional value than fresh because they're frozen so quickly after being picked.

Go Dry & Don't Use All the Spices

I can think of a few herbs and spices I see in recipes that are totally obscure. White pepper is my biggest pet peeve. I refuse to spend $4 on a tiny bottle of fancy pepper. I always substitute for regular pepper.

That's why I didn't write a cookbook. I don't make recipes and there are no pictures of recipes in here because I rarely follow recipes 100%.

You don't have to have a fully stocked spice cabinet, a few commonly used spices will do. Over time you'll figure out the seasonings you like and stay true to those. There's no point in wasting $100 on a cabinet full of spices you've used maybe twice.

We can all agree that fresh tastes better but store-bought fresh herbs and spices are way too expensive for a tight budget. Try growing your own. But I'll note, for the sake of personal experience, if you're consistently killing them, stick to dry.

You can find a variety of inexpensive dried herbs and spices at ethnic markets. They usually come in bulk so I suggest going with another frugal friend and splitting the cost and quantity. Tiny mason jars or reusable empty spice jars are a great way to store them.

Choose Your Organics Wisely

I'm not personally convicted to buy all organic produce, but for those who are and are simultaneously trying to lower your food budget, there's hope and a strategy.

You've probably heard of the "Dirty Dozen" when you're trying to eat organic on a budget. These are the fruits and vegetables with the highest concentration of pesticides. Either buy these organic or avoid them altogether.

MEAL PLANNING ON A BUDGET

If you're giving up all or some of the Dirty Dozen, you can replace them with the "Clean 15." These are fruits and veggies with thicker skins that protect the edible part from pesticides.

You'll have to make some sacrifices on organics if you want to tighten your grocery spending, but by being strategic you can satisfy both goals.

Minimalist Couponing

Couponing gets a bad rap but if you do it right you can save some money. The way most people muck it up is by spending too much time on it. We relate couponing to binders full of coupons, stacks of newspapers, printers going at all hours, and long waits in the grocery store line.

I don't buy many name brand things, thus I would be buying a lot of things I don't need with all those coupons. I'm all for getting the most bang for your buck so I follow two simple rules for what I call "Minimalist Couponing."

First, I only clip coupons I know I'll use for sure. I don't leisurely look through coupon books debating on whether I "could" use a coupon. I rapidly go through these things and only stop when there's a brand I know and love or have been wanting to try.

The same goes for Ibotta. Ibotta is an awesome app that gives you rebates (gives you money after your purchase instead of saving it upon purchase) for specific items. It's mostly name brand but there are always rebates on some generics so I'm all for it. But I don't "claim" rebates on products I'm not going to buy. I scroll through the app quickly and only "claim" what I'll use.

I use it because there are always a few "any item" rebates that can be used on store brand items like milk, bread, or just having a receipt from a certain store (I got

25 cents just for buying something at Walmart yesterday.)

Second, I won't go out of my way. I will go the extra mile to find a compatible manufacturer coupon for coupons in grocery store ads, but I'm not going to print 50 and go to five different grocery stores to maximize my stockpile. This is the method the people on TV use to get $700 worth of groceries for free. My time is better spent making money versus saving money on products I may never use!

It's a lot harder to do this nowadays but the fastest way to find stackable coupons is to look at your store's coupons first (the coupon shouldn't say "manufacturer's" anywhere on it), and then search the internet for a matching and compatible manufacturer's coupon. Don't search all day, The Balance has conveniently put together a list of the best websites for coupons, so if it ain't on one of those, don't waste your time.

Shopping at Aldi

Alright, this is the part of our program in which you can skip to the next chapter if you're physically unable to shop at Aldi or if you've shopped there for years. Basically, if you live in the Midwest, Pacific Northwest, Northern California, or Louisiana, I'm sorry for your loss, see you in Chapter 4.

For everyone else...
In my experience, the best way, by far, to save money on groceries is shopping at Aldi. The prices are a fraction of those at other grocery stores, the quality is way better than other discount stores, and its small size allows me to shop at lightning speed to avoid "off-list" distractions.

Everything about Aldi is designed to help home cooks on a budget.

That's why I meal plan and modify recipes to accommodate Aldi's selection. Aldi has 90% of what I want so it's not worth going to multiple stores and risking the temptation of seeing something else I "need" to follow a recipe completely.

I know Aldi can be intimidating for people who don't shop there regularly. If you have the pleasure of living or shopping near an Aldi, I want you to have the confidence to shop like a pro by the end of this chapter.

After you read this you'll be prepared to make your grocery list, tackle all five of Aldi's aisles with finesse, and check out with ease. Let's get started.

Understanding Aldi

Aldi cuts corners on service to give you quality products at half the price of the other guys. If you asked me to pay extra to have someone bag my groceries, arrange produce beautifully, or return my cart for me I'd say no every day. That's essentially what you're paying for at bigger grocery stores, the price is built into products.

Aldi erupted in Germany after World War 2 when people didn't need that fancy stuff, they just needed food they could afford. So Aldi has smaller stores, less selection, no bags or baggers, and makes you return your own cart so they can save on labor costs.

But don't worry, Aldi offers some of the best hourly wages among its competitors, a 5% 401K match, paid holidays and, at least at my local store, the employees seem to like their jobs. Aldi streamlines everything for its employees, from displaying products in the boxes they came in to having a ton of barcodes on products so they don't have to hunt for them at checkout.

All this makes shopping at Aldi cheap and really fast.

Most Aldi locations are open 9 am-9 pm Monday through Saturday and 9 am-8 pm on Sunday. Opening later and closing early is another way Aldi saves on labor costs and keeps prices low.

Aldi Locations

Aldi has 1,700 as of writing this and plans to have 2,500 stores open by 2022. Aldi is also actively remodeling its current stores. You can find a store near you and future grand openings on [their website](#).

If there's a new Aldi opening nearby or a "grand re-opening," you should definitely attend the event. There are free gifts, tastings, limited release products, and it's the only time you can get a legitimate Aldi coupon.

Before You Go

Aldi has two types of weekly ads. The official Aldi weekly ad is mailed to houses near its location, so if you get one in the mail or newspaper it's likely you're close enough to shop it. The weekly ad has produce picks, meat specials, and other seasonally selected sales. I like to look at the ad before I meal plan but you can count on most of the sales being on in-season items so it's not always necessary.

Just like other grocery stores ads, not every item in Aldi's weekly ad is on sale. Be on the lookout for the words "New Low Price." That denotes that an item is truly on sale. Most sales in the ad run Wednesday to Tuesday.

The in-store ad is called Aldi Insider; it's full of limited availability Aldi Finds. Mostly non edible stuff but there are a few Specially Selected food products in there too. I find that all of Aldi's products are good quality for the price you pay. If you see something you've needed, it's definitely worth getting it at Aldi when it becomes available.

It's not uncommon to see a line form outside of Aldi on Wednesday mornings because of the limited quantities of Aldi Finds. We've purchased some big things like a workshop toolbox, patio set, and air mattress from Aldi, and all are better quality and lower price than the best deals at Walmart and Target.

You can find both the weekly ad and Aldi Insider online up to two weeks in advance. Advance notice is great because it gives you plenty of time to plan for those Aldi Finds.

Bring Your Bags

Aldi doesn't offer bags like a normal grocery store; it's another time and cost-saving method, so bring your own reusable bags. If you forget bags, you can also use any empty boxes you see around the store, but it's a lot easier to bring your own than to hunt those down.

Have a Quarter Handy

Shopping carts require a quarter deposit. There's a contraption on the right side of the handle that you push a quarter into and the lock pops out, allowing you to pull your cart out. To return your cart, you stick that metal lock in the back side of the doohickey and it pushes the quarter out the front.

You can always tell an Aldi noob by the way they're fidgeting with the cart lock, so now that you know, you won't look like a noob.

Sometimes you'll catch someone unloading their cart and you can trade them a quarter for their cart. Other times there are good Samaritans who will pass their cart along to you and not want a quarter in return. I always like to keep the chain going if I can. It creates a special feeling of connectedness that's hard to explain and probably sounds weird if you've never experienced it.

Navigating Aldi

Aldi specializes in making the basics affordable. You'll find a lot of specialty items at Aldi but they're seasonal. There are some items you can always expect to find. This is a short list and based only on my experience at my local Aldi.

The layouts of all Aldi's are a little different, older ones are set up like a maze while newer stores are more free flowing. Regardless of the order in which you shop, here are the main sections you'll hit and the good stuff to look for in each.

Produce

All the produce, in my experience, has been fresh and long lasting. There's always a variety of apples, oranges, berries, and lemons. There are several exotic fruits available when in season like mangoes and pomegranates.

There's always a wide variety of vegetables from celery, onions, sweet peppers, potatoes, and carrots. Seasonal produce includes watermelons in the summer and squashes in the fall/winter.

Check out the organic section to find prices leaps and bounds cheaper than Whole Foods.

Frozen

Frozen corn, asparagus, broccoli, and peas are always available, and seasonal mixed vegetables change throughout the year. Aldi's ice cream is SO GOOD and thankfully available year round. If you see the Peanut Butter S'mores, you have to try it. It's divine.

Every Wednesday in our house is pizza night. And by pizza, I mean Aldi brand Mama Cozzi's Four Cheese Frozen Pizza. We add olives to it and each take a half. I've grown to prefer it to greasy take out pizza. Our usual Pizza Hut order comes out to just over $8 with a coupon, but we're satisfied with our $3 frozen pizza.

If you're really looking to splurge (and by that I mean spend $5) you can get the extra large Take & Bake pizza in the refrigerated section. The five-cheese pizza is AMAZING. I don't know what the fifth cheese is but it makes all the difference. It's bigger too, so you can have a slice or two for lunch the next day.

Refrigerated

Check your eggs for cracks before you take them. I've been pleased with all dairy products, especially the gourmet cheeses. Aldi's milk doesn't last as long as other stores so don't get the gallon unless you're going to finish it before your next trip. I get the organic milk and it's worth the money. It tastes better and it's not very expensive.

Pantry

I've never bought a bad pantry item or canned food item from Aldi. There's a great selection of canned beans and vegetables, the Italian and Mexican sections are great, and you can get all your baking needs there too.

Grains are limited to rice and quinoa, and dry beans are limited to black and navy. While the selection leaves much to be desired, the quality has always been good.

Aldi Beer & Wine

Out of the way, Trader Joe's, Aldi has the wine game on lock. Aldi's brand of wine, called Winking Owl, is good but they have some even better wines that don't even break $5. Burlwood Pinot Noir is my favorite. They also have wines rated in the high 80s-90s according to Wine Spectator.

Aldi has a limited but good selection of beer. I like the Broegel Bock and Kinroo Blue Belgian White. Not every Aldi carries beer and wine but if yours does you should definitely compare it to your favorite brands. I think you'll be pleasantly surprised.

Aldi Gluten Free

LiveGfree is Aldi's gluten free brand and it's one of the most affordable out there. The brand includes everything from frozen foods and snacks to pantry items. I'm not gluten intolerant but when I see a liveGfree product on sale, I'll get it because it feels healthy.

Checking Out

Checking out is basically the same as any other store but goes way faster. Cashiers swipe items and put your items directly into the cart, then you'll switch your cart with the new one. So don't attempt to take any of the lonely carts you see by the registers, they're there for a reason. There's an area at the front of the store for you to bag your groceries. Once you've paid you just pull your cart over and fill up.

In March 2016 Aldi started accepting credit cards, and in September 2017 started accepting Apple Pay and Android Pay. Aldi also accepts EBT but does not accept WIC or personal checks.

Aldi doesn't take manufacturer coupons and Aldi store coupons are like unicorns, most of the time they're fake but once in a while they're real. This is true at grand openings and re-openings where you can get $5 off $30 coupons.

Aldi vs Walmart

It used to be that Aldi had significantly lower prices than Walmart. But Walmart has caught on and their prices are pretty similar now. According to the most recent price comparison I found on Don't Waste the Crumbs, it's still cheaper on most items, just not by much.

You can compare weekly ads from both in your area to

be sure. So even if you don't have an Aldi near you, you can still get great prices at Walmart. I live near both and, while Walmart is actually closer to me, I choose to go to Aldi.

I choose Aldi for two reasons, first reason being that it's faster. Walmart is big and crowded and I could spend as much time waiting in line as I do shopping. When I shop at Aldi I'm in and out in 30 minutes. A list helps speed things up but there are some time sucks you can't control at Walmart.

The other is quality. I find the produce and dry goods to be much better at Aldi vs. Walmart. I can let produce from Aldi sit in my fridge for weeks (whoops) but by the second day after a Walmart trip, the produce has already gone bad.

But if you're someone who needs certain things from Walmart that you can't get at Aldi, you really don't need to make trips to two different stores to save money.

Action Steps:

- Find out what fruits and veggies are in season.
- Look for coupons in current ads and check for stackable coupons.
- Find an Aldi near you and check it out.

[3]

MEAL PREPPERS

I'm not the world's greatest cook and I don't love cooking, so there are countless other things I'd rather do than play chef every day. The problem is, I can't afford to eat out every day and I don't want to eat prepackaged food all the time with all its hidden sugar, salt, and additives.

And the thing is, you can use all the planning and grocery saving techniques in the world but if you don't make that food, you've wasted more money than you've saved.

That's why I believe meal prepping is as integral to saving money as meal planning and smart grocery shopping.

Meal prepping doesn't have to be all about reheating leftovers. That's a boring way to live if you ask me. You can use a variety of methods to make fresh meals *and* save time during the workweek.

It does take some pre-planning though. Luckily for you, I love planning enough for the both of us. I'm not perfect (hey, sometimes Sundays are for napping) but since I've implemented weekly meal prep, there's been a big improvement in the number of meals I prepare during the week and a decrease in the food I throw away.

So if you struggle in this area, I hope these tips will help you as much as they've helped me.

Schedule It In

You'll typically need 30 minutes per recipe to prep, which for five recipes is two and a half hours. I'd schedule three hours on whatever day you choose, to account for set up and clean up.

Scheduling this on your calendar should make it non negotiable. I like to do it as soon as I get home from the grocery store, but the beauty is you can do it at any time, night or day.

You might also go over three hours on your first few prep sessions. Soon you'll get a feel for how much fits in what container and you'll be organized enough to remember which recipe you're chopping that onion for, but for now, it's ok to be a little slower.

Don't make a habit of meal prepping all day, enjoy your relaxation time. Once you've been doing it a few weeks, cut yourself off at three hours. You might not get everything done but the time crunch will inevitably make you a faster prepper and keep you from dreading it.

Sort Ingredients by Recipe

When you have all your ingredients, the easiest way to stay organized is to sort them by recipe. By having everything out for a recipe, you can determine what size container you'll need for it and easily switch from one recipe to the next.

There might be some overlap in ingredients but you'll figure out by the end what goes where and you'll do it a lot faster with organization.

What to Have

Parchment Paper: Parchment is the one roll every kitchen should have. It's a nonstick cooking and freezing liner that is useful for all things. I'm passionate about it.

Aluminum Foil: While I prefer parchment for baking and freezing because it's non-stick, foil forms a great insulated barrier for meat in the freezer. If I'm short on parchment I'll use foil in the freezer.

Wax Paper: Wax paper is coated with wax, making it especially good for freezing things on, as they will peel right off. But don't put it in the oven. Wax melts; take it from someone who learned this the hard way. If you're looking to limit the clutter in your kitchen drawers, I'd say stick with parchment and foil.

Gallon and Quart Freezer Bags: I use gallon size for full meals and quart for individual ingredients. I'll also put unused quantities of store bought frozen produce in a freezer bag to preserve freshness. Plastic zip freezer bags are a staple for meal preppers because they're easily labeled with a sharpie and they freeze flat for bulk storage.

Cutting Boards and Knives: You probably have these but it may be time to upgrade. If your cutting board has deep grooves or knife cuts then it's time for a new one. Bacteria can get caught in there and that's a recipe for disaster. A few dishwasher safe wooden cutting boards are all you need. Wood naturally resists bacteria better than plastic and the dishwasher is the best place to sanitize.

Glass Containers: For leftovers or anything you'll microwave later, use glass storage containers like Pyrex.

Pyrex isn't my favorite because the lids crack easily but I have a few favorites on Amazon you can see in the resource guide for this book.

Plastic Containers: Ideally we could all afford nice glass containers for everything, but plastic is better on the wallet. I also prefer to travel with it because I'm a klutz. I reserve my plastic containers for non-microwave stuff because microwaving plastic can release BPA and phthalates into your food (especially fatty foods like meat and cheese) disrupting the endocrine system. Needless to say, if you're going with plastic, buy BPA free.

Rimmed Baking Trays: These are essential for roasting veggies and freezing individual ingredients. Rimmed trays in different sizes (I have three) are good for fitting into small spaces and holding veggies and meat on different trays.

Sharpie: LABEL, LABEL, LABEL. Bags should be labeled with the meal or ingredients and any cooking or special instructions. If I'm putting it in the freezer I also write the date it was put in there.

3-in-1 or Instant Pot: When we got married, we got a gift that we hadn't registered for but changed my life. It was a 3-in-1 slow cooker, rice cooker, and steamer. I used to have just a slow cooker and made burnt rice on the stove. With this one appliance I haven't burned rice since.

You don't need a 3-in-1, but it makes things go a lot faster, especially because you can steam veggies and cook rice at the same time. You can see the one I have in the resource guide.

Another appliance that's all the rage right now is the Instant Pot. This is definitely a progression appliance and you don't need one starting out. I got one recently to experiment with and I still find myself reverting back to my old 3-in-1 most of the time. I'm a creature of habit.

Chop What You Can

Most veggies can be pre-chopped on Sunday and will last all week or longer in airtight containers. It's especially advantageous for veggies that require some extra prep, like eggplant, which needs to be salted prior to cooking in order to eliminate bitterness.

Softer vegetables like tomatoes and cucumbers will lose their crispness after 3-4 days. If you really want to avoid extra chopping and clean-up, eat your BLTs and cucumber sandwiches at the beginning of the week.

I don't personally pre-chop apples and avocados but you can always use a little lemon or lime juice to keep them looking fresh longer.

This is also a great activity for couples to do together. Travis isn't as fast in the kitchen as I am but he can chop vegetables as well as anybody, making prep time go quicker and we get some sweet quality time together.

Store What You Can Where You Can

The containers you store your ingredients in can also be used to store leftovers after cooking, so keep future hot foods in glass containers and sauce or salad ingredients in plastic. That's fewer dishes, for the win!

You'll need more containers up front because food has more volume when it's raw. I also store garlic and onion separately from the rest of the dish because they typically get sautéed first. I store as many vegetables in reusable containers as I can but I inevitably end up using gallon zip bags when I run out or don't have big enough containers.

Label your ingredients by recipe and/or quantity and sort them by ingredient for easy access. Washed and dried lettuce keeps best in sealed plastic gallon-sized bags, and chopped onion should be kept in a fridge drawer on low humidity.

If you don't have much fruit you can put it in that drawer, or change your veggie drawer from high to medium humidity to prevent your whole fridge from smelling like onions.

We'll talk more about food storage and preservation in the next chapter.

If in Doubt, Freeze It

I don't typically get uncomfortable prepping for six days at a time in the fridge but some people feel you shouldn't do more than three. If that's you then you can still prep for the week, just pop meals for later in the week in the freezer.

Another method I use is making a double batch of a recipe I know I like. I'll use one during the week and save the other for later. Ready-to-slow-cook freezer meals are a lifesaver on Mondays when I didn't have time to go to the grocery store the day before.

My best experience with freezer meals has been with the slow cooker. Most oven meals don't freeze well and some take 48 hours to defrost (mine were still frozen after 24). Most people only do meats in their slow cooker, but I find it's fantastic for soups and pretty much anything you can put over rice.

That being said, don't put frozen raw meat in your slow cooker. Raw meat will sit at an unsavory temperature for too long and risk spoiling. Also, if the recipe calls for dairy, don't put it in your freezer meal. Milk, cream, and cheese should be added near the end of cooking to avoid curdling.

You might also want to freeze individual fruits and veggies to keep them longer. We'll talk about this more in the next chapter but for now here are a few tips for freezer meal success:

- To freeze foods that could stick together like burgers, bananas, and mangoes, freeze them flat on parchment-lined rimmed baking trays overnight, then put in freezer bags.
- Gallon and quart sized freezer bags are best for freezer meals because you can label them with a sharpie, remove most of the air within, and cut them to easily remove the contents if still frozen.
- Seal freezer bags most of the way and use a straw to suck out remaining air. This is highly advised for long-term storage (up to six months is safe to retain flavor).

If you're still hesitant, here's Greatist's list of 19 foods that keep well in the fridge and how to prep them. Start with these foods and you'll see how easy it is to prep for a week at a time and keep produce looking fresh.

Bulk Roasting

If you want to cook everything on meal prep day, one of the hardest things to do is cut down oven time. So many things, so many temperatures. Here's a quick reference guide to help you know what items go in the oven together:

- Very Low, 250-275 F: Slow roasts and braises.
- Low, 300-325 F: Cakes, veggie and chicken casseroles.
- Moderate, 350-375 F: Pot roast, most roasted vegetables, quiche, and muffins.
- High, 400-425 F: Quick roasts, baked and roasted potatoes.
- Very High, 450 F: Bread and pizza.

Reheating Leftovers vs. Cooking Every Day

Some people prefer to cook everything on meal prep day and portion it out to reheat all week. Others, like me, prefer to prepare everything and leave the cooking for the day of.

Each has its pros and cons. If you cook everything on meal prep day, you'll spend more time prepping but you'll only need to press a few microwave buttons to make dinner later. Alternatively, leftovers are usually not as good as a fresh meal.

Cooking every day is tiring and sometimes you don't even have 30 minutes to eat food, much less prepare it. And then there's always the day you forget to take your freezer meal out to defrost or you forget to put it into the slow cooker.

So, in my house, we have both on hand. Even if I have a recipe scheduled, life has a way of not cooperating. For those nights I know I can make a simple sandwich and heat up a can of soup.

Things don't always go the way we plan and one of the keys to making it work is flexibility. Don't fall into old habits of running to a restaurant or ordering through UberEats, commit to eating what's in your fridge and you'll see a significant difference in your spending.

Action Steps:

- Schedule your prep time.
- Make sure you have all the necessary tools.

- Pick a recipe on your meal plan to double for a freezer meal.

[4]

REDUCE, REUSE, EAT

I included this chapter mostly for me. I've been planning and prepping, batch freezer meal making and slow cooking for years now and while I've found all kinds of ways to save on the food that comes into my house, I've been ignorant as to how to get the most out of it.

In personal finance we like to talk about not just making money but making your money work for you. You can do the same thing with food. There's no way to use 100% of what you bring in, but you can make the most of what you have.

There are four ways to reduce your food waste:

- Limit what you buy.
- Store it in a way that extends its freshness.
- Preserve it for later use.
- Find an alternative use for it.

This chapter goes hand in hand with meal prepping, we want to make sure we're not saving all this money just to send it to the garbage the next week. I'll go through these food waste prevention tactics in order of importance and desirability, so if you don't have a ton of time you'll get the most important stuff first.

But hey, you made it this far, might as well finish, right?

Limit What You Buy

Go in with a grocery list and avoid impulse buys. Tired of seeing this one? Get used to it.

This still leaves room for the one time in a million that Aldi has jalapeños but they're not on my list. You better believe I get them. But I make sure to plan a meal for them once I get them home. I'll usually add an extra day to the bottom of my menu for it.

It's why "Reduce" is the first part of "Reduce, Reuse, Recycle"—you save the most money and throw away the least amount of the things you don't buy.

How to Store Your Food for Max Freshness

Did anyone ever tell you what those drawers in your fridge are for? Do you know there are parts of your refrigerator that are colder than others? These are all things I didn't know until recently, and I'm willing to bet I'm not the only one.

If you're spending all this money on groceries and buying them at discount stores or CSA's where they're known to have a shorter shelf life, then it'll greatly benefit you to know how to store your foods so they're fresh for as long as possible.

To start, your fridge should be set to **40 degrees Fahrenheit or lower,** but not low enough for ice to build up. This is the most energy-efficient way to run a fridge (yay for saving money on the electric bill too).

The **bottom shelf is the coldest** place in the fridge; keep raw or defrosting meat, poultry, and fish here. Keeping meat on the bottom also keeps it from accidently contaminating other food in the fridge if it leaks. You can be even safer by storing raw meat in a clear plastic bin or container.

Upper shelves are slightly warmer, good for leftovers, drinks, dips, and yogurt. If you want something (without raw meat) to defrost slightly faster, the top shelf is a good place for it. The **door is the warmest** part of the fridge and is great for storing condiments.

There are typically three drawers in the fridge: a **cheese drawer** that keeps cheese and butter from absorbing smells and tastes of the other food inside the fridge, and two humidity drawers.

These humidity drawers, also called crisper drawers, have always perplexed me. I keep my notches in the middle because I have no clue what they do, besides keeping loose apples from rolling around in the fridge. Sure, I could've Googled what they're for but who has time for that?

Well, friends, turns out they have a purpose, and a pretty important one at that.

Those drawers have a vent that regulates airflow in the drawer. The high humidity setting closes the vent completely. This reduces airflow and increases the humidity in the drawer. The **high humidity drawer** is good for fresh herbs, strawberries, and most veggies, particularly those that wilt (like leafy greens).

The **low humidity** setting opens the vent letting air flow freely through the drawer. More airflow is good for ripe fruit (except strawberries) and avocados because they emit ethylene gas (involved in the natural process of ripening). Mushrooms, peppers, and other veggies that tend to rot quickly should also be kept in low humidity to preserve their life.

Alternatively, once I chop greens and veggies, keeping them in airtight containers also keeps airflow out so there's no need to keep them in the drawer at that point. And I don't typically prep fruits (other than strawberries) unless they're in overnight oats because they go downhill so quickly once cut. The drawers work best if they're at least two-thirds of the way full, so let that be your encouragement to fill your fridge with fresh produce!

Some produce doesn't need to be refrigerated, and actually do better **on the counter.** Bananas, garlic, onions, potatoes, oranges, pineapple, grapefruit, tomatoes, and unripe fruit all last up to a week outside the fridge.

Pro tip: Don't store potatoes and onions together. They both emit gases that speed up the ripening of the other. Store potatoes in a paper bag to keep this from happening. I like those hanging produce baskets to keep everything ventilated and out of the way. You could also use a big bowl to keep everything in one place.

Have Easy Emergency Recipes

Every week you'll have two nights with no assigned recipe. These are meant to repurpose leftovers, raid the pantry, or use up produce on the brink of going bad. And sometimes you'll just be too tired to make your planned meal. For those nights you'll need emergency recipes.

Emergency recipes are easy go-tos for making a new meal with old ingredients. Monday's roasted veggies taste better in a quiche on Friday, those extra potatoes could be a hash if you throw a fried egg on it, and stale cereal makes a legit crust for chicken and fish.

Identify your favorite herb and spice combos and keep a few sauces that are good on everything. I like salt, garlic powder, paprika, smoked paprika, and cumin. Even if you're eating the same vegetable every night, different sauces and spices will keep you from noticing.

My Favorite Emergency Recipes:

- Soup
- Parfait
- Wraps
- Frittata
- Smoothie
- Fried Rice
- Pasta Salad
- Infused Vodka
- Veggie Burgers
- Breakfast Hash
- Pickled Veggies
- Stale Chip/Cracker/Cereal-Crusted Chicken or Fish

Classic Flavor Combos:

- Garlic + Lemon Zest/Juice
- Garlic + Basil, Parsley, or Rosemary
- Garlic + Onion + Ginger (Great stir-fry base!)
- Sage + Rosemary + Thyme
- Paprika + Dill
- Lime + Coconut + Chili Flakes

Canning & Pickling

Have you ever canned before? It can be very intimidating. But if you do it right, you can store cheap produce at peak freshness on your shelf for up to a year. And with the rise in popularity of mason jars, you may have everything you need to can without having to buy a kit.

The easiest way to can is to use the water bath canning method. It can only be used for foods high in acid (pH below 4.6) like jams, jellies, marmalades, or whole fruits. Tomatoes can be canned but you'll have to add ¼ tsp of citric acid or 1 Tablespoon of bottled lemon juice to each pint to bring them to the correct pH.

There are many recipes for canning on Pinterest so be sure to use an updated recipe. A lot has changed in food safety since your grandma was canning and botulism is no joke. Here's a great video on how to can with a water-bath and a step-by-step guide to water-bath canning.

If you have vegetables you're unsure how to use, then look no further than our great friend, the pickle. Brining fresh vegetables in vinegar removes the need for a pressure canner and delivers a snack that's delightful. And you can pickle ANYTHING.

There are two methods for pickling: one involves a water bath, exactly like canning, and the other is known as the quick pickle, made in the refrigerator. The first preserves the pickles to be shelf stable, as if you were canning them, while the other makes delicious pickles that are good for about one month in the fridge.

In either method, this works best with fresh veggies so I recommend canning and pickling with in-season produce that's really cheap.

There are videos and guides on canning and pickling available on the book resource page at Modern Frugality for easy access.

Freeze It Good

If you ain't got time for canning and pickling, then freeze it. Freezing food is my preferred method for preserving food and is almost completely foolproof.

Freezing individual ingredients isn't much different from assembling freezer meals. While freezing takes away some of the crispness when thawed, you can prevent that by blanching. This is a highly recommended step for freezing vegetables.

Blanching partially cooks vegetables using boiling water or steam. It's an extra step that makes a big difference in the color, texture, flavor, and vitamin potency of the food. There's a video on blanching in boiling water in the resource guide. It's not as essential for fruit but still recommended by some.

Here's a guide to blanch times for some excess-prone vegetables:

- Asparagus: 2-4 minutes
- Broccoli (1-inch pieces): 2 minutes
- Cauliflower (1-inch pieces): 3 minutes
- Celery: 3 minutes
- New Potatoes: 3-5 minutes
- Onions (Quartered): 4-5 minutes
- Peas in Pod: 2-3 minutes
- Sliced Carrots: 2 minutes
- Summer Squash: 3 minutes
- Whole Baby Carrots: 5 minutes

After vegetables are done boiling, drop them in an ice bath long enough to stop the cooking process, then dry and divide. Instead of packing everything into one big bag, I like to pack them in portions common to most recipes. Seal the bags almost completely and then use a straw to suck out the remaining air—the frugal chef's vacuum sealing.

To ensure your freezer is working optimally, don't freeze more than two to three pounds every 24 hours. Your freezer works most efficiently when it's full, but contents still need room for air to circulate between them. I tend to freeze last week's vegetables when I'm prepping the current week's meals.

When freezing meat, portion it into usable amounts and place it in labeled and dated freezer bags. Suck the excess air out of the bags and wrap them individually in foil (also labeled and dated). Meat sealed like this will last about three months.

The best way to thaw frozen food is to move it to the refrigerator. Small bags will thaw in 24 hours; gallon bags will take 2-3 days depending on how full they are. When incorporating frozen ingredients into meal prep, there's no need to thaw before using. The ingredients will usually sit with the fresh ingredients in the fridge long enough to thaw before you need them.

Use Food Scraps

Sometimes, while searching the depths of my fridge, I'll find a forgotten avocado or a lone potato that's not worth using. Life's too short to force bad produce down your throat. You can use the non moldy parts of produce in a variety of ways.

There are a few ways to find lost food a new purpose. Foods like lemongrass, celery, avocado, and potatoes can be regrown from scraps. If you use these foods frequently and have the patience (and the green thumb), try growing them.

Or keep scraps in the freezer until you have a few cups and make your own vegetable broth for soups, grains, chili, etc. Good scraps for homemade broth are:

- Onions Peels
- Celery Leaves
- Mushroom Stems
- Carrot Peels
- Broccoli Stems
- Garlic Skins
- Greens on Their Last Leg

This saves you plenty on store-bought broth. Minimalist Baker has my favorite recipe for making your own vegetable broth but the simple story is that boiling onion, carrots, celery, a gallon-sized freezer bag full of scraps, and eight cups of water will get you a preservative-free broth you can use for anything.

Feed the Dog

Not all garbage disposals are in the sink, some walk around on four legs. While not a go-to method for reducing food waste, feeding safe leftovers to Fido is better than trashing them.

If you can save a few dog meals a month by replacing them with leftover sides or unused ingredients you were going to throw away, you might save yourself the cost of a bag of dog food as well. But you need to know which foods are safe and which ones to skip.

Good Foods:

- Cooked chicken (not bones, save those for homemade chicken stock)
- Cheese (watch out for lactose intolerance)
- Cottage cheese
- Carrots
- Plain non-fat yogurt
- Pumpkin
- Eggs
- Green beans
- Cooked salmon
- Cooked sweet potatoes
- Sliced apples (make sure there are no seeds)
- Oatmeal

Foods to Avoid:

- Avocado
- Chocolate
- Caffeine

- Citrus
- Coconut (including oil)
- Nuts
- Onions
- Garlic
- Raw meat
- Salt and salty snacks
- Anything with xylitol

And don't think I've forgotten about all the cat lovers. Cats can enjoy all of the foods dogs do, including lean beef and lamb, and should avoid the same foods listed above. Stick to individual foods versus leftover meals. You wouldn't want to feed your dog some chicken casserole only to later remember there were onions in it.

Compost

If you decide to grow a vegetable garden or regrow some of your most used veggies, then composting is a great way to save unwanted food from the trash and increase your chances of not killing your plants. And so many random things can be composted.

A compost is a one-to-one combination of dead leaves and branches (high in carbon) and veggies (high in nitrogen). This mixture gets mixed and moistened over several months, creating a nutrient-rich natural fertilizer for your garden. Fall's abundance of leaves makes it the perfect time to start composting for the spring planting season.
Also, fear not, small space dwellers, if done right a composting bin shouldn't have an odor.

Here are some common items you might otherwise throw away that you can compost, and items that should stay out.

Nitrogen Rich Items:
- Grass Clippings

- Vegetables
- Fruits
- Kitchen Scraps
- Egg Shells
- Tea Bags
- Coffee Grounds

Carbon Compost Items:
- Leaves
- Straw/Hay
- Wood Shavings
- Bark
- Pine Needles
- Sawdust
- Paper

What Not to Compost:
- Meats
- Grease
- Oils
- Pet waste

You'll need a 3' x 3' bin near a water source at least two feet from the fence or house. If you're living in an apartment or have limited backyard space, a small metal or plastic bucket or storage bin with a lid will work.

Water and stir your compost every week or two and it'll be ready to incorporate into your garden when it's dry, brown, crumbly, and gives off no heat. Add 4-6 inches of compost into your garden in the spring or add to water for several days and strain off to make your own natural liquid fertilizer.

There's a comprehensive list of things you can compost, what category they fall into, and special instructions for composting them.

Action Steps:

- Organize your fridge for better food preservation.
- Write down your favorite emergency recipes (and make sure you have the staples for them).
- Find a quick pickle recipe for a veggie that's on sale.

[5]

SAMPLE MEAL PLAN WITH PREP GUIDE

The problem I find with "made for you" meal plans is that a lot of them don't take into account personal tastes, seasonal sales, and the time I have to execute them. I've seen plans that have chicken in every meal and grocery lists with ingredients I'd have to go to three different stores to complete.

The meal plans that save you the most money and please everyone in your family are the ones you make yourself. But even with all this info it might still be intimidating to start. I want to give you an example of some weekly plans to get you inspired.

These sample plans still require a little work on your part. It's specific enough to give you new ideas and vague enough for you to tailor to different sales and palates. There are no specific recipes, though they're all easy to find via a quick Google or Pinterest search.

You'll see the meal plans aren't meat centric or strictly vegetarian, they're sale centric. Produce tends to be cheaper than meat so there's a lot more of it on a budget-focused meal plan.

I included as much variety as possible while sticking to low cost items. I'm one to get bored easily so I can't live off beans and rice forever. These are real examples of sales from weekly ads throughout the year at my local Aldi. Since most sales are seasonal, they'll be similar to sale combinations you'll see at any grocery store.

I've also included suggestions for prepping your meals. The idea is to have everything done on prep day so you can finish off and cook with little to no extra dishes. I hope these ideas give you ideas that expand your culinary horizon and save you loads of time during the week.

Week 1

This week's sales: Yellow squash, zucchini, green peppers, and chicken drumsticks.

Breakfast: Mini egg frittatas & overnight oats.

Lunch: Leftovers, but when you don't have enough for a full meal, add a salad with avocado, pepitas, and cherry tomatoes or a PB&J.

Dinner:

1. Grilled zucchini boats (there are a variety of recipes for fillings) with drumsticks
2. Spaghetti with sauce made from canned tomatoes (and you thought pasta couldn't get any cheaper) and salad
3. Slow cooker soup and salad
4. Stuffed peppers
5. Chickpea curry with leftover veggies and chicken from drumsticks with rice

For overachievers: Squash and zucchini actually make yummy quick pickles.

Meal Prep

Make all breakfasts for the week on Sunday, put leftover veggies from last week into muffin tins and then pour in one egg per muffin, whisked or whole, your preference. Leftover or on sale fruit and nuts are great in yogurt and steel cut oats. Make sure you have the fixins for emergency lunch salads or sandwiches.

Cut and carve your zucchini, then make your filling. Put drumsticks in any marinade you want. Once you cook the chicken and assemble your leftovers during the week, any extra cooked chicken can be made into a chicken salad or added to the chickpea curry. Homemade spaghetti sauce is cheaper and healthier when made from canned tomatoes and herbs so no need to prep on that one.

A slow cooker soup can be pulled from your freezer or assembled in a bag and dumped in when ready. If assembling on prep day, prepare everything except dairy and leafy greens and put it all in a bag labeled with any additional instructions for cooking and serving.

You can stuff peppers with a variety of fillings. If ground beef isn't on sale or in your freezer, try brown rice and red beans. Prepare the filling and cut off pepper tops on prep day. Make extra rice to go with the chickpea curry. Add curry ingredients to a bag or container and add any extra green pepper, zucchini, and squash to stretch it.

Week 2

This week's sales: Tomatoes, white mushrooms, red potatoes, and boneless pork butt.

Breakfast: Avocado toast if avocados are on sale and a sweet quinoa porridge.

Lunch: Leftovers are still lunch but I'll get different salad toppings, maybe a hard-boiled egg, gorgonzola crumbles, and chopped asparagus. You can add bacon if you have it.

Dinner:

1. Slow cooker or Instant Pot pork butt with red potatoes
2. Margherita pita pizzas
3. Mushroom & potato tart with salad
4. Slow cooker chili
5. Caprese grilled cheese with salad

For overachievers: Try canning extra tomatoes.

Meal Prep

Avocado can be made into a spread or sliced throughout the week but you can make the quinoa porridge on prep day and portion it out for the week. It actually gets better as it sits. If it gets dry, mix in a splash of milk before you eat it.

Marinate the pork butt and cut and season red potatoes. Slice tomatoes and mozzarella for the pita pizzas. The tomatoes will keep as long as you use them within three days. If you have any leftover sauce from last week's pasta, this is the perfect place to use it. Slice mushrooms and potatoes for the tart. Spring for premade puff pastry for the tart crust. Still fancy with none of the time-suck.

Chop all your chili ingredients, cook meat if using, and store in a Tupperware with the onion separate. Alternatively, you can put everything into a ziplock bag and freeze it. Any extra veggies and pork after lunch leftovers can go into your chili. If there's no meat on sale, don't fret, vegetarian chilis are delicious, cheap, and make large batches. I highly recommend one that uses chipotle chiles in adobo sauce.

Slice the fresh mozzarella for the grilled cheese. Fresh is best and very affordable at Aldi. Since you're using these tomatoes at the end of the week, I'd wait until you're cooking to slice them.

Week 3

This week's sales: Pineapple, blueberries, strawberries, cucumbers, and ground beef are on sale.

Breakfast: Healthy blueberry oatmeal muffins and strawberry banana green smoothies.

Lunch: In addition to leftovers, have a spinach salad with strawberries and balsamic vinaigrette.

Dinner:

1. Burgers w/ sweet potato fries
2. Tacos
3. Blueberry & brie grilled cheese
4. Falafel in pita with tzatziki
5. Slow cooker stew

For overachievers: Quick pickle cucumbers and try your hand at a blueberry glaze for brisket or short ribs (whenever they go on sale).

Meal Prep

Bake muffins and freeze non-liquid smoothie ingredients in quart sized freezer bags. Season and form burgers, you can freeze leftovers for later. Chop and prepare taco ingredients. You can precook ground beef or crumble it for day-of cooking, depending on your time restraints.

Fruit and cheese go together like Chip and Joanna Gaines. You can use any sale fruit and cheese combo between two slices of crusty bread. Slice the cheese and fruit as needed. Falafel is easy to make in a food processor, stores well in a glass container, and just requires a little scooping and baking on the day of. Tzatziki is a cucumber yogurt sauce that can be made in the food processor once you clean out the falafel, in a blender, or even with an immersion blender.

A stew is a thick soup. Most people are familiar with beef stew, which is great if beef is on sale or you have some in the freezer. If not, ribollita is a delicious Italian vegetarian stew and there are plenty of chicken stew recipes out there. Chop and assemble all your non-liquid ingredients in a container or put everything in a ziplock bag and pop it in the freezer.

Week 4

This week's sales: Onions, celery, carrots, and whole turkey.

Breakfast: Breakfast sandwiches like McDonald's, only better, and baked oatmeal round out our breakfasts.

Lunch: Leftovers with a salad. If you're tired of lettuce (which I am, every few weeks) try a grain salad with buckwheat, wheat berries, or barley.

Dinner: Around holidays take advantage of seasonal sales. It'll take several days for a whole frozen turkey to thaw so you can either make an early trip to the store or reserve this meal plan for a week when you're not sick of turkey.

1. Turkey tetrazzini
2. Slow cooker vegetable soup
3. Turkey shepherd's pie
4. Asian stir fry
5. Turkey club sandwich

For overachievers: Make a batch of vegetable stock or freeze quart-sized mirepoix bags (fancy French word for the carrot, onion, and celery mixture that's the base for most soups).

Meal Prep

Put the turkey in the oven in the morning and let it cook as long as it needs. Give it time to cool before you start tearing it apart. Make the filling for the tetrazzini, put it in the casserole dish, and cover with foil. Wait until you're ready to bake to sprinkle bread crumbs on top.

Celery, onions, and carrots are the base for all great soups so this is the perfect week to make a big batch of vegetable soup. Cut up all veggies and store in a container until ready to go in the crockpot. If you have enough scraps to make a broth, this is a great time for that as well. It can be made in about an hour on the stove or 30 minutes in an Instant Pot.

Shred the turkey and cut the veggies for shepherd's pie and make the mashed potatoes. Keep separate until cooking. Cutting the stir-fry veggies is the only prep for that meal, and putting aside some turkey for the sandwiches is all you need for turkey clubs. You can precook bacon or wait until dinnertime to cook it, based on time restraints.

Action Steps:

- Write your own meal plan!
- Plan out your meal prep.

[6]

KEEPING IT REAL SUSTAINABLE

It's time to spread your wings, butterfly. Meal planning isn't the most exciting thing you could be learning on the weekend but it pays off. Think about every penny you're saving at the grocery store going toward your financial goals. Whether it's paying off debt, saving for your dream trip, or catching up on retirement, this one change can get you there faster than any other.

I mentioned batch planning as a way to keep meal planning sustainable but there's more to sustainability than just planning. Eating at home and keeping it affordable is a lifestyle you should be able to sustain forever. There are more tips that didn't fit into the previous chapters but are the cornerstone to ingraining frugal food habits.

Eat Smaller Portions

There's a simple solution to spend less on food—eat less. Easier said than done though, right? There are a few habits you can adopt to trick your brain into eating less.

Ditch the "dinner" plate and eat off smaller plates. We tend to clean our plates and our eyes are always bigger than our stomachs, so by switching to smaller plates and getting up for seconds (instead of keeping food on the table), you'll end up eating less.

It also helps to fill lunch containers up before serving dinner, then you know you'll have enough to fill you up the next day and it's easier to have a healthy snack at home later than to find one at work tomorrow.

Limit Fridge Raiding

Plans are just novel ideas if you don't stick to them. And a good plan can be completely derailed by fridge raiding. Eating tomorrow's lunch as a midnight snack only ends in going out for lunch the next day.

If you or a family member have a history of constant snacking that's affecting your grocery bill, then it may be time to have a talk about why. Of course, there's a line between normal and destructive snacking, teenage boys and athletes eat a lot, but everyone in the family needs to be on board with the budget.

Fixing this could be as easy as changing out pizza rolls for jerky or avocado. Snacks high in protein or healthy fats will fill you up faster and longer and get your grocery budget back on track. Otherwise it might be a matter of increasing self-control, which isn't my subject matter but is necessary to identify and work through.

Delete Your Food Delivery App

Food delivery is super popular with millennials. It used to just be pizza, but now you can get almost any restaurant meal delivered to your door for a small fee and tip. But not only do those delivery fees and tips add up, the ease of access tricks you into spending more.

When you're ordering from a menu without the piercing eyes of a cashier on you and no one waiting in line behind you, you can think about how nice that appetizer or dessert would taste with your meal.

Eliminate the convenience of ordering food from home or work. Take your credit card number out of the app and delete it.

Alternatives to Cooking

While a well stocked pantry can provide ingredients for quick emergency meals, there are just some nights you won't feel like putting anything together.

Luckily, eating at home doesn't always mean you have to cook. I could live off canned soup and steamer vegetables from the frozen foods aisle. Ready to bake meals at the grocery store can be a little more expensive but are still a fraction of the price of going out to eat.

Don't make it a habit but don't feel like a failure if you're heating up something from a can or package for dinner.

Painting the Town Green

We don't get out much, and I'm proud of that. We've been eating at home so long I don't know the names of most restaurants that have opened in the last two years.

If I do go out, it's a treat and I want to enjoy myself. I don't want to pick the cheapest restaurant with the cheapest entrée or settle for just an appetizer at a nice restaurant. Sharing a meal is a great idea but with our opposite food preferences there's no chance of Travis and I sharing something. So there are two ways we can splurge without spending our hard-earned cash.

First is asking for gift cards for birthdays and Christmas. For some reason my family doesn't understand the concept of wanting cash to achieve greater goals, they want to see me unwrap something. So we've accepted defeat and ask for gift cards to specific places, usually restaurants. We schedule our nights on the town so we can enjoy them versus using them to avoid cooking when we're tired.

Second is mystery shopping. There are many mystery shopping companies and they all specialize in different industries. My favorites for restaurants are A Closer Look and Coyle.

Mystery shopping is good for people with a high attention to detail and who enjoy writing. You're given a maximum reimbursement and as long as you spend under that, your entire check is reimbursed. Sometimes you even get a small payment on top of that.

If you commit to not spending money on eating at restaurants, then you'll become more and more resourceful and find you can enjoy a night on the town without spending much money at all.

Go Where the Free Food Is

National holidays like Cow Appreciation Day at Chick-fil-A and Free Pancake Day at IHOP give free meals with no purchase necessary. You can get free food on your birthday by signing up for emails (make sure to filter them out of your inbox for the rest of the year) and at supermarkets, either at grand openings or Saturdays at bigger stores.

Know when free food events are happening around you so you can put them in your meal plan.

If you don't live near chains that offer free food then don't fret, you're probably in a great area for foraging. Foraging is an adventure through the forest, picking wild produce.

You shouldn't start foraging without researching seasons, locations, and talking to local foragers. But once you get the hang of it, you're not just saving money and adding interesting produce to your meals, it's a fun and free activity to do with friends.

Done-For-You Meal Plans

In the event that you just can't manage meal planning, then there are entire businesses created around meal planning for you. A lot of them offer a free month or two weeks, which is great to get into the swing of meal prepping without worrying about planning.

And some of them are very customizable, allowing you to eliminate foods you don't like, decide the number of meals you want every week, and input your nutritional goals. All my favorites have an app and include custom grocery lists for every meal plan.

Some programs I like and the reason I like them:

Cook Smarts: The Whole Package. Customizable based on diet, you can change recipe serving sizes, menus are designed to reduce food waste, includes weekend prep instructions, and teaches you how to cook every meal. Only offers four recipes per week but at $6-$8 per month it's a great value for all it encompasses.

eMeals: Most recipes. Twenty-eight different meal plans based on diet, offers seven recipes per week and allows you to choose the number you want to cook. When I used it I found the vegetarian meals pretty average. And there's no way to customize a low carb vegetarian meal plan. If you don't care about customizing, then this plan might be a good pick for you, coming in at $5-$10 per month.

PlateJoy: Best recipes. Fully customizable based on diet, batch cooking and slow cooker options, focused on reducing food waste, with interesting and tasty meals.

PlateJoy recipes often include unique ingredients that aren't available at Aldi and don't take sales or meal prep into consideration and costs $8-$12 per month

Final Words

Most of the time I don't know how it all works out. But it does. The funny thing about planning is that life rarely goes according to plan. Every week something will come up that wants to derail your budget, but you'll get better at diverting those budget busters.

Take the time to learn the art of meal planning and cooking and you'll create frugal food habits that will transform your spending in areas far beyond the grocery store. Committing to a life of cooking at home can sound boring at first, but my favorite memories have always been with friends and family around a dinner table, not in a restaurant booth.

So here's to spending less money, living more years, and never passing up the opportunity to learn something new. Cheers!

IF YOU ENJOYED THIS BOOK CHECK OUT JEN'S OTHER BOOK:

The No-Spend Challenge Guide

In The No-Spend Challenge Guide you'll learn how to use No-Spend Challenges to reach your financial goals faster and transform your spending habits to finally be able to stick to a budget. You'll discover:

- Why budgeting alone isn't working
- The psychology behind your impulsive spending
- How to pay off debt fast while still having fun
- Ways to do for free what you've probably been wasting money on
- Ways to save money on your financial obligations
- How to make the most of your time without spending money

Whether you're paying off student loan debt, saving for your first home, or just trying to control your spending; This is a personal finance book you'll return to again and again. Click here to learn more & buy on Amazon.

Want More?

Get weekly stories about frugality in real life and motivating debt payoff stories at: www.modernfrugality.com

Made in the USA
Middletown, DE
29 August 2019